Calorie Counting
Healthy Eating
By Cathy Wilson

Copyright © 2013

Income Disclaimer

This book contains business strategies, marketing methods and other business advice that, regardless of my own results and experience, may not produce the same results (or any results) for you. I make absolutely no guarantee, expressed or implied, that by following the advice below you will make any money or improve current profits, as there are several factors and variables that come into play regarding any given business.

Primarily, results will depend on the nature of the product or business model, the conditions of the marketplace, the experience of the individual, and situations and elements that are beyond your control.
As with any business endeavor, you assume all risk related to investment and money based on your own discretion and at your own potential expense.

Liability Disclaimer
By reading this book, you assume all risks associated with using the advice given below, with a full understanding that you, solely, are responsible for anything that may occur as a result of putting this information into action in any way, and regardless of your interpretation of the advice.
You further agree that our company cannot be held responsible in any way for the success or failure of your business as a result of the information presented in this book. It is your responsibility to conduct your own due diligence regarding the safe and successful operation of your business if you intend to apply any of our information in any way to your business operations.

Terms of Use

Calorie Counting
Healthy Eating

By Cathy Wilson

Table of Contents

Introduction

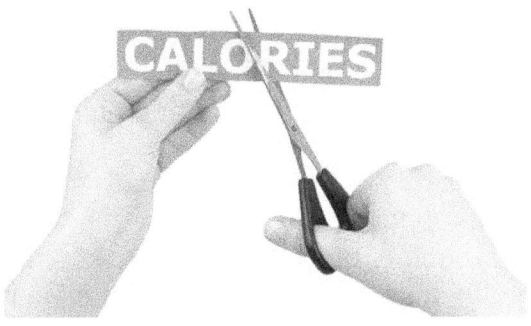

Getting healthy is downright confusing! One day you've got a big list of foods that are fantabulous for your body. And the next thing you know, experts are switching gears.

Suddenly all those pomegranates you've been patiently preparing, really aren't loaded with free radical fighting antioxidants!

To eat eggs or not eat eggs?
Are milk and milk products really just made for babies, and interfering with your good health?

Who do you believe?
BEST MOVE - Continuously arm yourself with *current* health and wellness information. And **COMMIT** to pondering **every** tidbit of information flowing through your spongy brain, with an open mind, and logical perspective.

You may have to dig deep from time to time for explanations. A pain in the *arse*, but necessary. For the most part, just follow your gut instinct and you'll do just fine! If it makes sense, and you've got the nutrition experts also giving you the thumbs up, then you're good to go, for now anyway.

My schooling, professional, and life experience for over 20 years, has been health; fitness and nutrition specifically.

I'm passionate about health and life.
With this introductory book, if you gain just one piece of useful information to help reach your weight loss goals, or help you look or feel better in any way, then I'm one happy camper!

With an open mind, searching for the positive, you **WILL** only get *healthier*.

In order to lose weight, it's pretty black and white. You need to eat fewer calories, and expend more energy. This means, if you're metabolic rate dictates you burn 2000 calories a day on average, you've gotta find a way to burn more than 2000 calories worth of energy consistently to blast fat over time.

PERSPECTIVE TIME - If you're going to lose one pound of fat, experts at *WebMD*, say you need to expend an extra 3500 calories on top of the number of calories you need to eat to maintain your weight.

So if you need 2000 calories to maintain your weight, you've gotta find a way to subtract 3500 calories over time, in order to lose a pound.

You can do this with a combination of less food and healthier food choices. Another option is to increase your physical activity each day.

According to *Healthy* Living, your best bet is to combine healthier eating strategies in smaller amounts, with regular intense interval muscle building and cardiovascular training regularly.

Think of it as killing two birds with one stone. Speeding up the fat loss process, and increasing the chances you'll sustain it!

Your mind is very powerful and influential in how you look, feel, and view life. Flipping your switch to positive helps blast fat, and gets you happy with yourself and life. That said, one stumbling block people get stuck on, is that **ALL CALORIES AREN'T CREATED EQUALLY.**

Not only does your body accept, breakdown, process, and absorb foods differently, each and every person is uniquely different in utilizing the exact same foods. Even as you age, your body deals with nutrient absorption differently.

In other words, Mary's body might process a Twinkie one way, with most of it contributing to her growing fat stores. Whereas Timmy's body might be so physically fit, and used to burning through calories, that a Twinkie's simple sugar energy's gone before he even has a chance to throw the wrapper out.

His body just utilizes fats and sugars more effectively than Mary's, even though a Twinkie is really not good for either of them.

Science says, eating too many of the wrong calories will make you overweight, then fat, and finally obese if you continue.

It's time for solutions.
Action plans that are practical and simplistic, for people like you and I to implement. The foods you eat shouldn't become your life focus. But it's important you're aware of how to make *better* choices, that'll help you lose fat, gain energy, deter disease, and flip your *life* switch to positive.

QUESTION - In general, do you opt for *good* calories or *bad* calories?

What are Calories

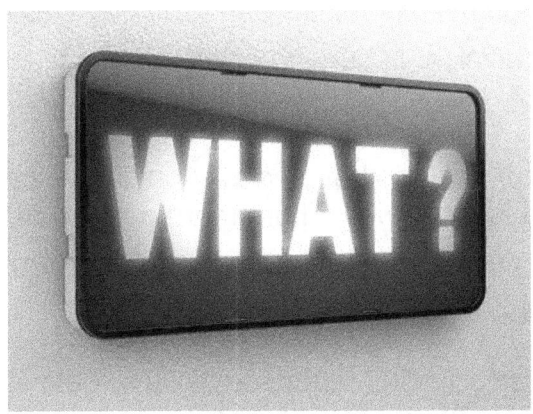

Let's start at the bottom of the barrel and work our way up. Let's understand what a calorie is, what it does for you, and why it's critical to lose weight for eternity.
You wouldn't be alive if you weren't consuming calories. Calorie is simply another word for energy. It's a recognition tool your body uses to understand amounts of energy you are consuming, namely foods and beverages.

Pointers to Ponder
*The foods and beverages you consume each day are based on calories and not energy
*Your body sees and understands energy as calories, a number from which to work.
*In order for your body to function mentally and physical, it requires calories.
*Your body is pre-programmed at birth to function optimally with a specific number of calories. Unfortunately your poor lifestyle choices, lack of exercise, *bad* calories food choices, and lazy tendencies, interferes with your

intrinsic needs, and screw up the way your body uses calories and stores them.

*There are calories in every single food you eat.
*Beverages that boast *zero* calories slip through the cracks, and have chemicals and toxins that make your body less efficient in burning calories normally. It's just like tying your legs together during a running race.

Perhaps *zero* calorie beverages should have calories because of this? You would burn more calories naturally, if you didn't put these chemicals into your system. It's something to think about.

Medical News Today, reports artificial sweeteners negatively affect your metabolism and insulin levels. Not good news if you're looking to lose weight and steer clear of developing diabetes!

Calories are used to explain any sort of energy when you think about it. If your tractor's on empty, it's not going anywhere anytime soon, if you don't give it some calories. Tractors don't eat *food* of course, but if you gave it diesel *calories* you're in business. If you want your bicycle to move, **YOU** have to give it calories in the form of energy.

By peddling, you're transferring energy from your body to propel the bike forward. In simple terms, you're giving calories to the bike to move it, which also happens to be a great cardiovascular activity to zap fat!

Same as anything in life, there's both good and bad. When you wake up, your energy stores are on zero, and it's important you provide body calories for your body to function optimally.

You could grab a pastry from the vending machine at work, and technically your body would work. Or your better choice is a healthy nutrient rich breakfast full of *good* calories; oatmeal with fresh berries, skim milk, and a banana works.

This gives you protein to build muscles and provide energy, complex carbs to keep your energy levels high longer-term, healthy fats to keep your thinking crisp and clear and provide energy, along with numerous essential vitamins and minerals to help your body function optimally mentally and physically.

Choosing a pastry gives your body the calories it requires to function. But not the nutrients it requires to function optimally, starve off disease, burn fat, strengthen immunity, and help you to think straight.

These simple carbs are loaded with *bad* fats. They're high in calories, have high sugars, and almost zero good nutrition. You're going to shoot your blood sugar levels through the roof eating a pastry, and back down to the bottom of the barrel before you can blink.

CIP - Cathy's Important Point - There is a difference in the *type* of calorie you fuel your body with. Do you want to run your tractor with premium diesel fuel, or with a nice dose of alcohol?

What happens over time, is your body will start *telling* you the *bad* calorie foods you've been feeding it, aren't wanted.

How does it do this?
It takes place in the form of lack of energy, increased aches and pains, fat gain, obesity, disease and illness,

more injuries, and your body will make it really difficult to enjoy and appreciate life in general.

My Thoughts . . .
The choice is yours.
Learn to open your mind and start listening to your body, or continue on your life path of living short of your true desires and abilities.

It's not about being perfect, or making sure every single calorie the goes into your mouth is good.

This book is about waking up and gaining perspective. Starting to make and understand better food choices and implementing. If you make just one better food decision each day, you're moving forward in a positive direction, towards losing weight and bettering yourself.
That's should be your focus.

Types of Calories

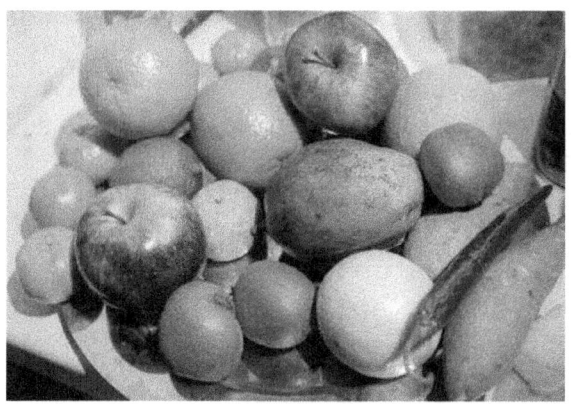

Calories are a universal tool that's used and abused, and then used some more. Many people believe a calorie is a calorie. That 200 calories of potato chips, is the same as 200 calories of fruit.

According to *Nutrition Today*, that's just not true.
We do know eating more calories than your body needs to function, leaves you fat. Too few calories results in weight loss. Considering the differences between types of calories, how your body works, and the *amount* of calories your body requires and utilizes, is the golden ticket to sending fat to *Neverland* forever.

Scientists know, if you consume excess of calories, they'll be stored as fat.
WHY?
By eating too much, you're COMMUNICATING to your system to build up energy reserves, for an emergency

situation. A point in time where you may not have access to food for a long period of time.
Your body only reacts to your physical actions!

This scenario was *VERY* real back in ancient times. But today the only emergency you might run across, is that your car breaks down and you have to actually walk to the restaurant. Rarely in our developed world is food not readily available.

Your body doesn't know all this. It's intrinsically programmed to be prepared for the worst. Your quest is getting your body to trust you and defect from nature, and the threat of disaster.

Mentioned previously, a calorie is a measurement used to qualify energy.
The three main kinds of calories are:
*Proteins
*Carbohydrates
*Fats

I don't care what you *think* you might know. Your body needs each of these calories in varying amounts, in order to function, fight off disease, and build your muscles and mind strong, to stand the test of time.

Scientists have researched these different calories inside out, upside down and backwards. If you don't agree with this information, you're going to have to take it up with all of them.

Each of these three kinds of calories burns up when your body heats them up or turns them into calories for use. They each have a different chemical makeup, and are found in different sources of food.

18

Protein

Proteins are the building blocks of life. Every cell in your body has protein in it. In measurement terms, protein has 4 calories per unit. This macronutrient in required by the body in larger quantities. It essentially consists of a whole lot of amino acids all connected together happily.
When you digest proteins, they're broken down into specific amino acids for use. There are 20 amino acids in total. We won't go into detail here, but it's important you know the basics.

Functions of Protein

*Help build muscle, repair tissue, and sustain cell health
*Provide energy for the body
*Helps structure your body
*Build bones, fingernails, skin, and hair
*Activates enzymes
*Moves muscles
*Transports enzymes through the body
*Assists with hormone communication
*Triggers blot clotting
*Regulates PH and fluid balance

Protein is something your body doesn't make or store, and this means protein calories must come from food sources. It's important for your good health to get adequate amounts daily for your fantabulous health. Remember approximately 50 percent of your body is made of protein!

Sources of Protein

In general, there are two main sources of protein; meat and non-meat sources.
MEAT SOURCES
-Beef
-Poultry
-Wild game meat

NON MEAT SOURCES
-Shellfish and fish
-Eggs, milk, and milk products
-Nuts and seeds
-Legumes

CIP - All protein calories aren't equal.
A complete protein food source has all 20 amino acids for your body to use. Non-Meat sources are not complete. This means you have to combine 2-3 in order to give your body all of the amino acids it requires to function optimally.

In other words, if you aren't eating meat for your protein source, you'll have to do a little more juggling, to ensure your body gets *EVERY AA* it requires to function and deliver.

In general, 2-3 servings of protein each day are required according to nutritionists, more if you're muscle training, or exercising intensely and often.

Carbohydrates
Carbohydrate calories are not created equal. Scientists agree, the *type* of carbohydrate you consume, is more important than the amount you eat. A simple example is, a cup of quinoa or a slice of healthy whole grain bread, are better calories for you than a serving of French fries or pastry.
Hence the confusion begins!

Carbohydrates Explained
You'll find carbohydrates in both healthy and unhealthy foods; pasta, rice, bread, pastries, milk, cookies, soda, pie, corn, sweet potatoes, and whole grain bagels. Most people choose carbohydrate foods with sugars, starches, and fiber.

Your body needs carbohydrates in order to stay strong and healthy. They give your body the glucose it requires for energy. The *quality* of carbohydrate you filtrate into your body, is important, because there are *good* and *bad* carb food sources.

Healthy Choices

Carbohydrates that are natural and unprocessed, prove to be exactly what your body craves and desires, to function with spunk for the long term. Included are healthy whole grain breads, whole wheat pasta and wild rice, sweet potato, various fruits, beans and other healthy vegetables, which deliver essential vitamins, minerals to optimize your health.

The fiber helps to remove harmful toxins, and antioxidants and phytonutrients to help protect your body from illness and disease.

Unhealthy Choices

These are referred to as simple sugar carbohydrates, which break down quickly in your body, causing energy to be short-lived. These carbs often overload your system with fast absorbing sugars, spiking your blood sugars, and driving your energy levels through the roof instantaneously. Problem is, what goes up, must come down! Included are white bread, pasta and rice, soda, cookies and crackers, cakes and pastries, sweets, and other treats we teach ourselves to crave.

Eating these *bad calorie* carbs in excess, will deplete nutrient sources, interfere with level energy, trigger diabetes, heart disease, depression, sleeping issues, and thinking problems, and all sort of other troublesome issues.

Keep in mind this manifests over time. Moderation is critical, and looking to make *better* calories choices should be your focus.

Perfect?
No. Just better choices.
FACT - 5-6 servings of *good* carbohydrates are suggested by the experts of *Healthy Living*, each day. 3/4 cup of oatmeal, 1 slice whole grain bread, 1 banana, 1 sweet potato, 1 cup of beans, and 3/4 cup of whole grain rice does nicely for the day.

Again diversity is key, with proper serving size. Particularly when you're battling that nasty fat of yours that chooses not to cooperate.

Carbohydrates measure in at 4 calories per unit, the same as protein. This means they offer the same amount of energy for your body, but each are utilized differently.

Fats
Welcome to the wild and whacked out world of fats. This is where the real confusion begins. I'm going to try and keep to the surface, so I don't end up confusing myself! You should actually be happy fat exists, because if it wasn't for fat, you wouldn't exist. Fat calories are essential for your body and mind to function. Problems arise in the crazy amount of fat we consume as a society, along with the kinds of fats we're partial to.

Just as there are *good calories, bad calories*, there are *good and bad* fats. Yikes!
Relax - Take my hand and I'll guide your through!

Benefits *of Fat*
*Provides body with energy
*Protects internal organs from injury

*Regulates body temperature
*Assists with essential vitamin and mineral absorption
Fats are made of oxygen, carbon, and hydrogen, in different combinations. This gives you the different types of fat on the market today. There's saturated, trans fat, hydrogenated, and unsaturated. Most people categorize them as healthy or unsaturated fat, unhealthy or saturated (trans) fat.

Trans fat is the worse, because it's a synthetic form of bad fat. So it's chemically altered for longer shelf life, more stability, better structure and color, and it's much cheaper for the manufacturers.

They choose to poison you and make more money.
Saturated Fat has the most number of hydrogen atoms possible in structure. These fats are found mainly in animal products, like butter and animal fat. Palm and coconut oil are also categorized here. I will say, coconut oil is the exception to the rule, cuz it's a saturated fat that's heart healthy, according to *Dr. Oz!*

That's another book in itself. Coconut oil fat has too many natural health benefits to name.

Saturated fats are usually solid at room temperature, and in large quantities over time, will mess up your internal systems, and cause serious health issues.

Unsaturated Fat doesn't max out in the hydrogen department. These fats don't come from animal sources. They're healthy and liquid at room temperature for the most part. Olive oil, sunflower oil, and almond oil, are examples of healthier unsaturated fat choices.

According to nutrition experts, we need less than 30% of our daily caloric intake from fat.

Most of us get fat from the foods we eat, condiments like salad dressing, and from our cooking methods. There aren't very many people in the developed world that need to worry about getting enough fat into their day. Most of us need to work on making sure we get the right *type*.

Choosing *good* fat calories is important in losing weight fat and getting healthy.
1-2 tablespoons of olive oil, 1/4 cup avocado, or 4-5 olives, are all considered a serving of fat, just to give you an idea.

By choosing to watch your serving sizes, eat a healthy and well-balanced diet, and pay attention to the fats you're eating, weight will come off, energy levels will rise, and you will begin to feel like you're on top of the world all over again.

VIP - Fat calories measure in at 9 calories per unit, which is more than double that of protein and carbohydrates. This also means, the more fat you eat, the fatter you'll get. Just look around if you need clarification.

If you want to make a change, you've got to commit to opening your mind and taking positive action. There's nobody to blame but yourself.

Stop your blaming and start getting healthy-happy.

My Thoughts . . .
Understanding the three different types of calories is important in the big picture. If you're looking to get slim and optimize your body function, you need to pay attention to what type of calories you're eating, and how much.

A measurement tool so you know how many calories you're munching down, and whether they're good *or* bad, is the only way you'll make progress. Time for you to give your body the calories it craves in the right amounts. Listen to your body, and learn how to fuel it well.

Your reward will be weight lost, and fantastic health.

Isn't it worth playing for?

How your Body Burns Calories

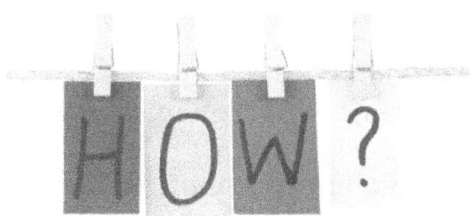

Just like no two people are alike, calories are different too. It's wise-owl smart to understand how your body takes in, breaks down, absorbs, and utilizes calories. This determines and reflects on your body composition, energy levels, bodily health, and life positivity.

If your body isn't burning maximum calories, you're not likely a happy camper. Understanding how your body burns calories, and creating a plan to burn more calories more efficiently, only makes you better as a whole.

Are you one of these people that blames your fat on a slow metabolism?
SHAME ON YOU!

Your metabolism is intertwined with your specific weight, but chances are it's not what you think. Your weight isn't normally reflective of a slow or lacking metabolism. For the most part, your extra fat is a direct result of the food and beverage choices you make and your daily exercise habits, or lake thereof!

The good news is, each of these factors are controllable. Better still, they can be altered to increase your natural metabolism, or the rate in which your burn energy or calories.

Whether you choose *good* or *bad* calories, is an integral yet important piece of this puzzle.

Your **Basal Metabolic Rate** is the rate in which your body burns calories, or uses energy at rest.

Factors that influence your metabolism are:

*Body composition, weight, and age
*Sex
*Overall health condition
*Lifestyle
*Genetics
*Exercise routine
*Eating habits
*Sleeping regimen
*How your body breaks down food

For the most part, your resting metabolism or basil metabolic rate doesn't alter much. About 65% of the calories you burn each day are used for this.

How Much You Weigh and Metabolism
Some people are always going to use their *slower than normal* metabolism, as an excuse for their fat rolls. Scientists, doctors, and medicinal experts across the board, say the majority of the time, that's hogwash.

Slow metabolism is not the reason you're fat. The decision not to do anything about it, is.

Even when people starve themselves, weight loss is going to be extremely difficult.

Why?
Your body recognizes you're depriving it, and literally slows your metabolism to conserve energy, while this *crisis* passes. It's a self-created miscommunication between your intentions and your brain or bodily needs.
When you don't give your body the nutrients it requires to function, it will fight back.

It doesn't trust you to feed it properly again. And in a panic burns energy as slowly as possible, storing every single carrot stick you feed it as fat for later use.
Bottom line is, if you want to burn fat and get healthy, you've got to encourage your metabolism to *want* to burn more energy and fat. Fuel it properly, exercise regularly, sleep properly, and make sure you choose *good* calories for the most part, and the trust between your body and self will re-establish.

At this point your body will forgive you for all the wrongs you've committed, and work *WITH* you to blast fat and keep it off.

The Key to Losing Fat is to get your Body to Burn More Calories . . .
How do you do this?

*Look to fuel your body with nutrient dense *good* calories in the right amounts
*Eat on a regular basis to keep energy levels up, and blood sugars stable
*Get quality sleep
*Focus on increasing your metabolism with exercise; muscle building, and cardiovascular exercise regularly

29

*Make better lifestyle choices to improve your overall good health

Eating plenty of healthy fruits and vegetables, provides your body with all the essential vitamins and minerals it requires to function optimally, fight off disease, and make certain you're strong from the inside out; mentally and physically.

Providing a constant flow of healthy calories into your body throughout the day, encourages a boost in metabolism. This means you've the energy available when your body needs it to perform.

Highs and lows throughout the day are pretty much abolished, and you're less likely to turn into Medusa. Your body needs calories to burn if you want to get rid of your pesky fat, and release untapped energy.

Psychology Today says sleep is something critical for fat loss and good health. Your body works hard, and needs a chance to fully recharge each and every night. If you don't let your internal systems rest and reload with energy, you're starting each day with half a tank of crappy gas, instead of loading up with premium fuel.

If you aren't getting a quality 7-8 hour sleep each night, you're bandaging your body, and eventually your wounds will become infected.

The best route to increase your metabolism is to exercise regularly. This forces your body to burn extra calories. And if you're eating plenty of good calories, lean protein, and good carbs in particular, your body will shine in the calories burning department, leaving you lighter and happier fast.

Muscle burns more calories than fat. This means strength training a few days a week to build lean muscle not only burns extra calories, but also builds your body strong to burn more calories even when you're sleeping. Interval training is what experts deem the fastest and most effective exercise regime to burn calories. Alternating periods of intense cardiovascular exercise at varying intensities, with set times of intense muscle building exercising, keeps your mind and body guessing, and burning a high rate of calories in a short amount of time. Diversity is key in increasing your calorie burn and rate of metabolism. Interval training sessions like boot camps, are the best route to achieve both.

45 minutes of cardio, 5-6 days a week, along with at least 15 minutes of weight or strength training, two days a week, is key to getting your body to burn for you. It's definitely a step in the right direction.

We all know there are lifestyle choices that don't help with your health. Smoking, illegal drugs, and even breathing in household and environmental chemicals, stresses your systems.

The toxins from these choices interfere with your fat loss efforts, the rate in which your body burns calories, and even with the absorption of the *good* calories you're trying to provide.

Any step away from these negative lifestyle choices, is a positive step in the right direction for fat burning and optimal health.

YOU MATTER!

My Thoughts . . .

Many blame their genetics, or metabolism for being overweight and unhealthy. It's time to change this thought, and understand there are ways you can rejig your thinking. Positive action to get your metabolism working harder for you.

Taking the time to fill your body with the proper amounts of good calories, exercising regularly, and making better lifestyle choices, are the first few steps you need to commit to, in order to change your reality.

If you want lean, energetic, disease-free and happy, you can have it.

*All you've got to do is **make** it happen.*
Use this information to build a happier you.

Calories Truths

It's true, if you want to alter your eating habits to lose fat and get healthy, you've gotta understand calories.

Here's some straight up factual information that puts calorie truths center stage.

TRUTH: Calories are the key to losing weight or gaining it.
You would think if you eat less calories than normal, you'll drop the weight lickety-split. Sorry to say, it's not quite that simple. You do need to cut your energy intake to lose fat. But what's more important, are the kinds of calories you're ingesting.

Calories aren't created equal, that's for sure.
If you decide on the right calories, you'll lose weight and not starve. Pick the wrong calories, and you'll still get fat, and your tummy will be constantly rumbling.

That's the truth.

TRUTH: JUST cutting back on total calories eaten, only delivers short-term weight loss. It's just not going to stick.

If only there was a mathematical-like instructional manual to lose fat! A list of exact and precise steps universal, for everyone to lose the exact amount of weight they choose.

Well, weight loss is a science, but it's also gotta be something you're willing to experiment with, to figure out works for you. It **HAS** to fit into your lifestyle, pay respect to your likes and dislikes, and preferences and tolerances, or you're barking up the wrong tree.

Research shows, most people trying to lose weight won't succeed. Many people start off on the wrong mental foot, by referring to it as *dieting*. It's a word that naturally has negative perspective, and most definitely isn't setting you up for success when change is so freakin tough to start.

Let's get back to the truth here. Cutting calories **WILL** work for a short while. Using the numbers initially and cutting back on calories, figuring there are about 3500 calories in a pound, will work for most out of the starting gates to lose fat.

Partially because you're unknowingly overeating to the extreme. Where any change in your unhealthy eating, will encourage weight loss. People do lose weight on a low calorie diet for the first few months, but then chaos usually strikes.

People often continue to lower the calories, until the body is forced into starvation mode. Where your metabolism drops, and your body tries to store every single calorie you eat as fat.

WHY?
Simply because it doesn't trust you to feed it, and your body is smart. It knows **EXACTLY** how many calories your body is pre-programmed to use and not die. By lowering the rate of calorie burn, it's trying desperately to starve off your impending death!

Extreme I know, but that's how you've forced your body to react.

Another road people take, is to eat the same low number of calories, and expect the same rate of weight loss. Well, your body's a pretty clever poker player. It doesn't take long to figure out what you're up to.

Your body internally adjusts, predicts how much energy you're using, and what you're eating, cuz it's got your patterns memorized. This allows your body to slip into efficiency mode or autopilot, and not work so hard.
If you don't at least change and diversify in the healthy foods you're eating, you'll hit a frustrating plateau naturally, and your actions aren't going to keep giving you results.

SOLUTION!
Diversify, keep both your mind and body guessing in your eating and exercise, pay attention to eating fewer *good* calories and connecting with your body, and you'll continue to drop fat to your healthy level. Easier said than done I know.

Truth: It matters where your calories come from.
When people decide to cut calories and lose weight, they usually are immediately successful, because any amount

of calories cut is a good thing to your body. That's the initial perspective anyway.

After you lose the first few pounds, your body and mind start paying attention to the type of calories you're eating.

Your Body Knows...
*That 200 calories from high-bad-fat, high calories, high sugar, low nutrient bad carbohydrate chips, is NOT good for your body nutritionally speaking.

*Eating 200 calories worth of high fiber nutrient rich whole grain bread, with a tablespoon of high-protein good fat peanut butter, is a better choice for your weight loss, physical, and mental good health.

Calories from processed, refined, high-fat foods, are much more likely to signal fat storage to your body. Eat these foods, and they'll settle nicely on your tummy, hips, thighs, and arms, and give you a double chin if you choose.

If you have a decadent processed saturated fat chocolate chip cookie, with the same number of calories as a grilled chicken salad with extra veggies, will they affect your body the same because they have the same number of calories?

If you're measuring in nutrient terminology, they aren't even close. If you're looking to lose fat, I'd bet the house, option two's going to help you zap fat.

A few things to consider . . .
Thermal Factor of Food
Basically there are some foods that use more energy to chew, process, and utilize for energy than others. You've

trained your body to master storing fat, using few calories to do so.

This means your body is conditioned to be on holidays when you're eating junky processed foods. The carbohydrate process is fairly simple in the big picture. Although complex carbohydrates trigger your body to use more calories to get the job done.

Protein is a tad more complex in nature, and uses more internal energy to break it down for use. It has to be transformed into carbohydrates during the process.

Blood Sugar Affect

Consider also, the effect of the foods you eat on your blood sugars. Simple carbohydrates are absorbed immediately into your blood, spiking sugar levels sky high temporarily.

Examples here are white breads, sugars and pasta and sweets. What this does is encourage your body to store fat, pack on the pounds, and still feel like your hunger isn't satiated.

On the flip side, if you're eating fibrous fresh fruits and vegetables, and lean protein, your body has to use ample energy to process, with less sugars, and a longer work time.

This means your blood sugars stay level longer, and your energy levels are there for the using. Since your blood sugar levels don't shoot through the roof, fat gain is less likely.

Research shows blood sugar levels are reflective of weight gain.

Truth: Keep a record of the calories you eat to help lose weight.
This is a forceful trick tested and proven beneficial. It's too easy just to eat something and conveniently forget you just ate two cupcakes, six cookies, and a handful of chips before supper.

We condition ourselves to eat emotionally, due to boredom, or because of stress. This means you're not consciously thinking when you're munching.
A concrete recipe for obesity and poor health.

By physically recording everything you eat, the evidence is right in front of you. All you've gotta do is look down, to see all the *bad* calorie choices you're eating. And by opening your mind to change, you'll start connecting the dots.

You may see for breakfast you ate two pastries from the vending machine, and a can of soda. Because you've written this down, you can absorb and accept your reality and make the commitment to change this learned habit. You'll consciously accept the past as the past and move forward. Choosing to eat whole grain bread with oatmeal and fruit for breakfast, instead of junk, and feel fantabulous about it for all the right reasons!

Of course this isn't going to happen overnight. But keeping a food journal helps you take the first steps toward better health, and continue on full steam ahead.

Truth: Consuming less calories will help you live longer.
Research shows, people that eat healthy and eat less, tend to live longer than people that don't.

GOAL - Give your body the number of calories it wants and needs, not too many and not too little, is what you should strive for.

Healthy Eating research studies show, people eating smaller amounts of *good* calorie diets, have lower levels of inflammatory proteins in their blood. This is a good thing, because these nasty proteins trigger just about every single disease and illness known to mankind. The more of these proteins you've got floating around your internal systems, the faster you're going down for good.

Truth: Your body has a pre-set optimal calorie range, where you function best.
This may seem a little weird, but you were born with an internal mechanism that had a set calorie range and weight range, where your body functioned optimally.

What happened?
Through time, most of us have majorly screwed this mechanism up with fad diets, starvation, and overdosing on processed high fat foods and calories. I *KNOW* you get what I'm saying here.
We essentially get fat and reset this safety mechanism repeatedly, at a new level much too high to be healthy.

What now?
By eating the right amount of good calories for your body and lowering your weight back down to your healthy zone for at least six months, you can reset your internal calorie-weight meter at this healthy weight.
This just means your body will start working with you, to help you keep your weight stable, because it recognizes this as your new *optimal* level for function.

In other words, when you get to this point, your body will be more forgiving, and you're going to be a heck of a lot happier.

The Ultimate Truth - How Many Calories Do You Need? (Good Calories of Course!)

Again, there are no two people that need the exact same number of calories to maintain their weight, or the same amount and intensity of exercising to lose weight. You are unique, and so are the calories you need, and at what rate you burn each different type of calorie.
Sorry to confuse you here.

What number of *good* healthy calories your body requires, is dependent on numerous factors:

*Body composition
*Age and gender
*Genetics
*Activity level
*Lifestyle
*Current health
*Eating habits or style
*How much weight you're looking to lose
*Attitude

Your metabolism is a reflection of the rate in which your body uses calories, both good and bad. Fact is, it's the amount and type of calories you eat, compared to the number of calories you burn that determines if your weight is going to stay level, plummet, or shoot to the stars.

Understanding your Basal Metabolic Rate or BMR, is a gynormous clue in ensuring you're getting the right number of calories your body requires for your intentions.

You are in change of ensuring that it's good calories you're getting. Which will make reaching your weight loss goals a heck of a lot easier.

The main factors reflecting your BMR are:
-Body size, height, and weight
-Body composition, flabby, or muscular
-Age and gender

Nutrition experts recommend using a formula to calculate your number. This can be done by your nutritionist, or you can do it yourself on-line quite readily. Understand this number won't be exact, but it is a great place from which to start gaining control of your weight and health. It's a fairly accurate measuring tool, where you'll be able to *see* progress, a natural motivator for you to want more.

My Thoughts . . .
Bottom line is, you need to make good *calorie choices in the right amounts, burning more calories than you are ingesting, if you want to be successful in weight loss.*

A combination of eating less, choosing healthy fan-tabulous calories, and increasing your daily physical activity to find your rhythm, are all positive action steps that'll direct you healthy, happy, lean and strong.
But only if that's what you CHOOSE to do.

Good Calories

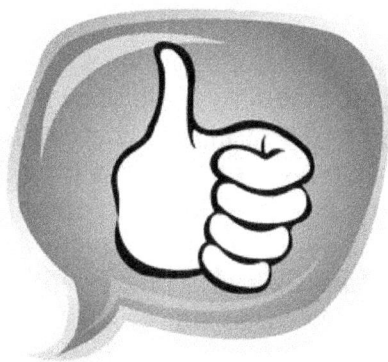

This is an introductory book. So I'm going to keep it simple, functional, and clear-cut right!

GOOD CALORIES are without interference, they aren't *fake* or processed, added or chemically altered. Good calories are the proteins, carbohydrates, and essential vitamins and minerals your body has required from the beginning of time, to function optimally.
These calories come from the foods you **know** you should be eating.

The natural wholesome foods that give you energy, fight off disease, regenerate tissues and cells stronger, strengthen your mind, ensure you stay at a healthy weight, and give your body exactly what it needs to work hard for you, and keep your motor running at a healthy pace.

Good Carbohydrate Calories come from . . .

Whole grain breads, brown rice, oats, and quinoa. Vegetables, beans, fruits, and whole wheat pasta are also
good carbohydrate calories. These foods give your body
the fiber it needs to get rid of harmful toxins. Along with
vitamins, minerals, antioxidants, and even some healthy
fats.

These diverse combinations, provide clean energy, fight
disease, keep blood healthy, help your internal systems
function with zip, and encourage crisp thinking.
Healthy Eating also says good carbs provide your body
with the glucose it needs to function optimally.

Good Lean Protein Calories come from . . .

Eggs, beans and legumes, lean beef, chicken and turkey,
fish, quinoa, milk products, peanut butter, nuts, seeds,
and veggies to start. Your body needs these 20 amino
acids present in complete protein to repair, build, and
maintain cells.

Protein helps transport oxygenated blood throughout
your body, build muscle, and keep your energy levels up.
Low fat is important, cuz the fat in most protein unhealthy, and interferes with maximum protein benefit.
Paleohacks reports it's often the toxins the animals eat
and are exposed to, that make animal fat harmful.

Good Fat Calories come from . . .

Vegetable oils, nuts, seeds, avocado, olives, and fatty
fish are great sources of good fat. These healthy good
calories are a great energy source, help you think better,
and protect your internal systems from physical damage.

My Thinking . . .

Good calories come from making healthy food choices in moderation. Even if you're eating too many good calories, they aren't good for you, if that makes sense.

By understanding what your body needs, making healthy food choices considering your goals, preferences, and tolerances, you'll succeed in blasting fat fast and reaching your true health potential.
BELIEVE IT!

Bad Calories - Empty Calories

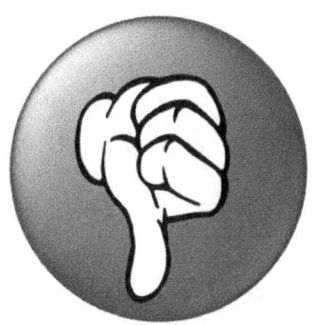

The flip side of the coin are nasty bad calories. They're the calories that make people obese, and full of disease and illness. These calories affect the mood negatively, messes up your mental, triggers depression, anxiety, sleep troubles, and all sorts of other unhealthy realities for oodles of people.

Bad calories long-term **WILL** result in bad health; lack of energy, extreme tiredness, longer recovery time from injury, more injuries, less patience, increased negativity, more chronic aches and pains, troubles sleep and waking, confused thinking, and serious illness.
Each of these are reflective of making bad calorie choices.

Choosing processed fast foods with loads of calories, bad fats, toxic chemicals, preservatives, lots of refined sugars, and many seriously damaging ingredients you can't even pronounce, **WILL** make you fat and unhealthy in time.

FACT - It's not a matter of *if*, but *how much* and *when*. In general, bad calories come from bad fat foods. Energy choices loaded with unhealthy saturated and trans fats. Fats your body has no use for, particularly in the crazy-butt amounts we eat them.

These fats build up in your system and literally slow you down, building up toxins because you have no way of shipping them out. Even if you did, it's next to impossible for your body to keep up with the demand to purge crap!

The result?
Obesity, disease, illness, and eventual death.
Bad Calories are found in . . .

*Fast Food - Processed hamburgers, fries, onion rings, cheesy breads, deep fried meats, and so forth.
According to *Livestrong*, a recent research study revealed fast food consumption had the biggest impact on obesity levels.

*Packaged Cookies and Cakes - These tasty bad calorie treats are usually loaded with seriously toxic trans fat, for longer shelf life, better taste and pleasing visual appeal. Just like photoshopping an image, except toxic.

*Boxed Foods - This includes toaster waffles, Danishes, and pancakes. Most of which have those nasty trans fat, lots of additives and preservative, and very few good calories.

*Microwave Popcorn - Place this in the same category as theater popcorn. Most varieties are loaded with harmful fat, that'll only add inches to your waistline.

*Frozen Foods - In particular, frozen dinners are extremely misleading when it comes to nutrition. Many are chalk full of cheaper trans fat, that poison you from the inside out. High in fat and calories, low in nutrition just doesn't add up.

You're better than this.
*Sodas and High Sugar Drinks - You've probably heard about the ridiculous amount of sugar in sodas today. Some have close to **TWENTY-FIVE** teaspoons of sugar in one can? Are you kidding me? That's as bad as my Starbucks lady friend!

These are empty calories that'll spike blood sugars and increase weight gain. In fact, sugary drinks are sort of like warming up for a race. They'll get your body *ready* to get fat. Bad calories to run far and fast from.

*Yogurt - Be careful here, cuz some yogurts are sweet-ened with *HIGH FRUCTOSE CORN SYRUP* to make them flavorful. HFCS is dangerous to your health, so be careful.

*Condiments - Although usually used in sparing amounts, many condiments are just nasty bad. Ketchup for instance, has HFCS that's only going to flip your fat calorie switch on, and invite the nasty squishy molecules in.

*Refined Cereals - Unfortunately, the big bad commer-cial world of advertising leads us to believe that *cereal* is always good for you. Problem is, that's pretty much a load of crap.

In fact, there are only a handful of *good* calories cereals out there. Even those with a few natural wholesome in-gredients, turn bad when excess sugars are added for flavor, and preservatives and other harmful chemicals for color and longevity.

Don't let the pretty packaging fool you!
BEST ADVICE - Take the time to read the ingredient list. If it's long, and you can't pronounce and understand what you're reading, don't buy it.

***Dressings** - Salad dressings are loaded with bad calories, and one in particular I'd like to pick on is ranch salad dressing. It has an ingredient Maltodextrin, that's just as bad for you as it sounds. When using dressings, use them sparingly, or not at all.

Nothing wrong with naked!
***Fried Foods** - These are high fat, high calorie foods with bad fats, cholesterol, and MSG to ice the cake. **NOTHING** about fried foods is good for you. Steer clear of fried foods, and you'll reduce your bad calorie intake.

***Chip and Crackers** - MSG and saturate fat should be enough to remind you of just how unhealthy these food choices are for you. They have no nutritional gain, and only bad calories to offer. These foods provide calories that love to stick to your legs, hips, tummy, and butt. I'll stop there.

***Sweeteners** - Sweeteners boast little to no calories, but unfortunately trigger so much turmoil to your health, that you're best to just call them bad calories, and steer clear.

Experts claim they can trigger:
-Depression and anxiety
-Insomnia and hives
-Serious disease, including Alzheimer's, diabetes, and blindness

***Cheese** - Most cheese is loaded with bad calorie saturated fats and sodium, none of which is good for your waistline or mind.

Processed Lunch Meats - They're chalk full of toxic chemicals and preservatives, unhealthy trans, and saturated fats. Again, these are bad calories all the way.

*Donuts, Pastries and Other Sugary Treats - All these tasty treats scream ALL BAD in the calorie department. Eat these, and you're asking for a few layers of insulation to be added to your frame.
My Thinking . . .

*Bad calories are not your friend, especially when you're looking to lose weight. They can be sneaky, and are often hidden, so you really need to know your stuff. Saturated and trans fat, sodium, chemicals, and preservatives, that are ample in these bad calorie foods, will leave you fat, frumpy, and depressed. Run far and fast from these **BAD CALORIE** foods, and you'll do well for yourself, mind, body, and soul.*

Pointers to Manage Calories

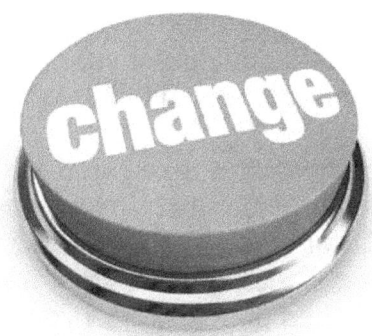

Now that you understand the importance of choosing *good* calories to fill your belly, it's time to open your mind up to strategies that manage your calories overall.
By understanding how your body works, what foods you should be eating, and in what amounts, you'll make it much easier on yourself, when it comes to running your calorie show.

Here are a few pointers to help . . .
*When eating out, do a little investigative research before you go. By choosing what you're going to eat before you get there, you'll increase the likelihood of controlling what you eat, and making good calorie food choices.

Many restaurant menus are available online. Or you can even give the establishment a call beforehand. This removes the unknown, when a decision needs to be made.

*Plan you eating at least a day or two before. Just knowing the foods you're going to eat, and having some of them ready prior to eating, removes some anxiety from the equation. Don't kid yourself, cuz life is busy, and often not knowing, will steer you straight back to your unhealthy and comfortable eating habits of days past.

*Understand the give and take relationship. You are only human. You need to cut yourself some slack. If you happen to go out with friends and overindulge on occasion, it's important to let it go. Hop right back up on the horse, even if you had dessert when you weren't planning on it.

SOLUTION...
Why don't you add an extra 30 minutes of cardio to your workout the next day, or reduce your food intake a touch? All this is going to do, is teach your mind that you're human, and get you back on track fast.
And you'll have even more motivation to make the *good* calorie food choices, in the *right* amounts.

*Measure if you need to. Until you're used to proper serving sizes, you may have to get out a deck of cards, to make sure you're eating just one serving of lean beef. Pour your whole grain pasta into a measuring cup, to ensure you're not giving yourself restaurant portions. This will help you stay within your calorie means, and learn to eat healthier effortlessly, with practice.

My Thoughts . . .

These pointers help you teach you how to eat within your means for your desired goals. Understanding that life is ever-changing, and so is your body function.
Diversify and enjoy, always aware of what you're eating, and how much. Making sure it's the good calories in the proper quantities on your plate!

Final Thoughts

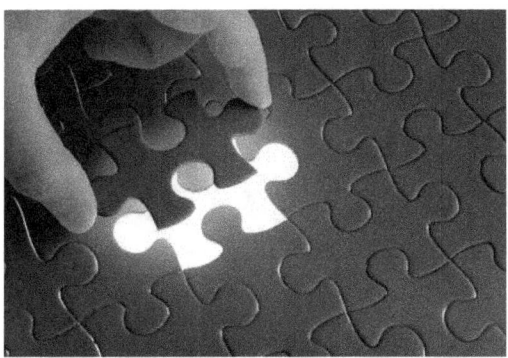

If you're going to succeed in blasting your spare tires, you're going to have to be honest with yourself. Lay all your cards on the table, and open you mind to change one manageable step at a time.

COMMIT to making better food choices!
If you think you can make healthy good calorie food choices for a few days, and maintain a significant weight loss, you might as well click your heels twice and go back with Dorothy to visit the tin man!

Getting yourself on track to lose weight sensibly and keep it off, takes GYNORMOUS changes in your eating. By recognizing, understanding, accepting, and implementing **good calorie** eating into your life, you **WILL** smash through each of your weight loss and health goals.

*Mind over matter here, and it's **YOUR** decision.*

You've got the smarts and basic knowledge required to slip your life switch to rainbows, cotton candy clouds, and bright sunshine.

TRANSLATION - You know how to eat smart, lose weight sensibly, and keep it off forever!
Don't you think it's about time to stop procrastinating and just get on with it?

Last Thoughts…

*THANK-YOU for reading my masterpiece. I hope you learned a little something, or at least got a few smiles.
*I would appreciate a millisecond or three of your time for a quick review, to help me build my masterful book empire higher.
*Whatever you do, don't forget to smile! And of course, check out my website for more of my e-Book masterpieces at: www.flawlesscreativewriting.com

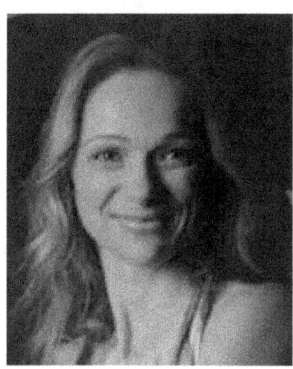

Cathy ☺